HERBAL SOLUTIONS FOR HEALTHY KIDNEYS

Complete Guide To Unlock The Power Of Nature's Remedies For Disease Prevention With Simple Herbal Approaches

DR. CHRIS FRIEDRICH

Disclaimer

This book on Herbal Remedies is intended solely for informational and educational purposes.

The content provided within this book is based on general knowledge and should not be considered as professional advice. The author is not a licensed medical professional, and the information presented here is not intended to diagnose, treat, cure, or prevent any disease.

Readers are advised to consult with qualified healthcare professionals before initiating any herbal remedies or making changes to their existing health regimen. The author and publisher disclaim any responsibility for any adverse effects or consequences resulting from the use of information contained in this book.

It's important to note that the content of this book is not endorsed by any specific platform or affiliated with any product or service.

The author does not receive any compensation or benefits from the promotion of specific herbal products or brands.

Readers should exercise their discretion and judgment when applying the information from this book, and they are encouraged to conduct further research and seek guidance from healthcare professionals to make informed decisions about their health and well-being.

CHAPTER 1
INTRODUCTION

Human health is a complex web that is finely knit, with different organs playing different roles in general health. Among these essential organs, the kidneys defend the body silently while carrying out the necessary function of removing waste and extra fluid from the circulation to create urine. Since the kidneys are essential for preserving the internal equilibrium of the body, it becomes crucial to understand renal health.

Synopsis of Renal Health

The kidneys are two bean-shaped organs that are located in the back of the belly. Their functions include filtering blood, eliminating waste, and controlling fluid balance. The kidneys' working units, called nephrons, put in an endless effort to guarantee that necessary materials are retained while hazardous pollutants are eliminated.

The filtration role of the kidney is only one aspect of its health; other functions include blood pressure regulation, electrolyte regulation, and red blood cell synthesis. Chronic kidney disease (CKD) and other renal disorders can interfere with these complex functions and set off a chain reaction of health problems.

The Need to Avoid Kidney Disease

Because renal impairment can have far-reaching repercussions, it is imperative to prevent kidney disease. renal failure is the result of chronic renal disease, which can advance silently and is frequently asymptomatic in its early stages.

The effects are not limited to the kidneys; they also impact bone metabolism, general health, and cardiovascular function. Furthermore, the necessity of renal replacement therapy and the financial burden of treating advanced kidney disease highlights the significance of taking preventative action to protect kidney health.

To stop kidney disease from getting worse and lessen its effects on people's health and healthcare systems, lifestyle changes, early detection, and efficient management are essential.

The Use of Herbal Treatments

Herbal medicines are becoming more and more popular as a natural and conventional means of maintaining health with the goal of holistic well-being. Herbal medicine has been used for ages to support kidney health in many different cultures. Herbal therapies are highly valued due to their ability to promote renal function, lower inflammation, and target the underlying causes of kidney illnesses. While scientific studies on the effectiveness of herbal therapies for kidney health are still in progress, some plants, like turmeric, dandelion, and nettle, have shown promise in laboratory tests.

Knowing how herbal medicines affect kidney function opens up possibilities for complementary and integrative approaches to modern healthcare in addition to drawing on traditional understanding.

In summary, it is impossible to overestimate the complexity of renal health and its enormous influence on general well-being. It is imperative to prevent kidney illness, which calls for a multimodal strategy that includes lifestyle modifications, early identification, and—interestingly—the possible advantages of herbal therapies. This introduction lays the groundwork for a more thorough examination of these ideas, which will delve into the intricacies of kidney health, the significance of preventive measures, and the developing role of herbal treatments in promoting renal health.

CHAPTER 2
UNDERSTANDING KIDNEY DISEASE
Structure and Purpose of the Kidneys

One of the body's most important organs, the kidneys, is crucial to preserving homeostasis. These bean-shaped structures, which are located at the back of the abdomen, filter waste materials and extra fluid from the blood to create urine.

Millions of nephrons, the functional units in charge of filtering, make up each kidney.

The kidneys receive blood supply from the renal artery, which helps with the filtration process. Then the blood that has been cleansed goes back into circulation via the renal vein. In addition, the kidneys play a role in blood pressure regulation, electrolyte balance, and the synthesis of erythropoietin, a hormone essential for the synthesis of red blood cells.

To fully grasp the consequences of kidney disease, one must have a thorough understanding of the complex structure and many activities of the kidneys.

Typical Reasons for Kidney Disease

Renal function can be impacted by both acute and chronic diseases, which can lead to kidney disease. Because diabetes mellitus is a common cause, excessive blood sugar levels over time can harm the kidneys. Another frequent cause that strains the kidneys' blood channels and reduces their functionality is hypertension.

The kidney's filtration system is impacted by infections, such as glomerulonephritis, which causes inflammation and damage.

A genetic condition known as polycystic kidney disease causes the kidneys to develop cysts, which impair normal kidney function. Adverse medication reactions, kidney stones, and autoimmune illnesses are among the other causes. Understanding the many etiological components is essential for efficient kidney disease management, diagnosis, and prevention.

Symptoms and Risk Factors:

It is critical to identify the risk factors linked to kidney disease to facilitate early detection and intervention. People who have diabetes or hypertension, or who have a family history of kidney disease, are at a higher risk. Susceptibility is also influenced by gender, age, and ethnicity. Kidney disease symptoms might appear gradually, thus awareness is important. Common signs include exhaustion, edema, variations in the color or frequency of urination, and ongoing itching. Complications including anemia and bone damage might develop as the condition worsens. Furthermore, people may develop hypertension and cardiovascular problems.

Healthcare providers can conduct timely tests and adopt preventative interventions by having a thorough understanding of these risk factors and symptoms, underscoring the importance of proactive kidney health management.

Addressing and managing kidney-related illnesses requires a comprehension of the complex architecture and functions of the kidneys, as well as a recognition of prevalent causes and associated risk factors and symptoms. This complex knowledge is essential for everyone who wants to protect their kidney health and well-being, not only medical experts.

CHAPTER 3
HERBAL APPROACH TO KIDNEY HEALTH
Historical Perspectives on Herbal Medicine

Herbs have been used medicinally for generations; many societies have included plants in their healing rituals. Ayurveda, Traditional Chinese Medicine (TCM), and Indigenous healing practices are examples of traditional medical systems that have long acknowledged the benefits of herbs for enhancing general health, which includes kidney function. These traditional methods offer a wealth of knowledge for the current investigation of herbal treatments for a range of illnesses, including kidney-related ones.

Fundamentals of Herbal Treatments for Healthy Kidneys

The foundation of herbal therapies for kidney health is an emphasis on the holistic aspect of health. Rather than focusing on specific symptoms, these treatments frequently try to bring the body back into equilibrium. The ability of herbs to enhance kidney function, encourage cleansing, and lower inflammation is taken into consideration while choosing them. For example, dandelion root is frequently utilized because of its diuretic qualities, which aid in the body's removal of waste. In a similar vein, turmeric's anti-inflammatory qualities are acknowledged for their ability to reduce kidney inflammation and improve overall renal health.

Herbs are frequently selected for their adaptogenic properties, which aid in the body's ability to adjust to stimuli and preserve peak performance. Adaptogens such as Rhodiola and ashwagandha have the potential to promote kidney function by influencing the body's reaction to stress.

It's also essential to comprehend how herbs function energetically in conventional medical systems. Herbs are classed in Traditional Chinese

Medicine (TCM) according to their energy qualities, which might affect their usefulness for kidney health depending on an individual's constitution. Examples of these qualities include cooling and warming capabilities.

Safety and Things to Think About

While using herbal medicines to support kidney health has potential, it's important to proceed cautiously and seek the advice of trained medical specialists when implementing these interventions. Potential interactions between herbs and drugs, personal sensitivities, and the caliber of herbal medicines are all safety concerns. If taken in excess, several herbs have the potential to cause unwanted side effects or interfere with kidney medicine. Furthermore, before introducing herbal remedies into their routine, people with pre-existing medical disorders or those receiving medical treatment should speak with their healthcare professional.

Ensuring the safety and efficacy of herbal remedies requires strict quality control. The authenticity of herbal products may be impacted by contaminants, incorrect identification of certain herbs, or differences in potency.

Potential hazards can be reduced by looking for goods from reliable suppliers and, whenever feasible, speaking with herbalists or medical professionals who are knowledgeable about herbal medicine. Additionally, continued study is essential to deepening our knowledge of the workings and effectiveness of herbal medicines for kidney health, which lays the groundwork for recommendations based on solid data.

The herbal approach to kidney health emphasizes concepts based on holistic well-being and is influenced by traditional methods.

For those considering complementary methods to improve kidney function, it is crucial to comprehend the background information, the tenets of herbal therapies, and safety concerns.

Although herbal remedies show great potential, their integration requires careful consideration, making educated decisions, and working in tandem with medical specialists to maximize safety and effectiveness.

CHAPTER 4
ESSENTIAL HERBS FOR KIDNEY HEALTH

A proactive strategy to preserve renal function is to incorporate important herbs into one's lifestyle. Kidney health is crucial for overall well-being. Because of its diuretic qualities, dandelion root is regarded as a beneficial herb for kidney health.

Its capacity to increase the production of urine may help remove toxins from the kidneys, thereby encouraging the best possible functioning of the organs.

Another essential herb for kidney health is chanca piedra, which has been utilized traditionally in many cultures for its ability to break down kidney stones and facilitate their removal. Given that its name means "stone crusher," it is fitting given its past application in treating kidney-related issues. This herb may help maintain the kidneys' normal functions and avoid the development of stones.

Nettle leaf is also known to have a beneficial effect on renal health. Packed with antioxidants, it could lower the risk of kidney disease by preventing oxidative stress. Nettle leaf also contains diuretic qualities that could help support the body's natural fluid balance and aid in the removal of waste.

The anti-inflammatory qualities of turmeric, a spice, are drawing notice because they may be beneficial to kidney function. The major ingredient in turmeric, curcumin, has antioxidant and anti-inflammatory properties that may help reduce kidney inflammation and shield the kidneys from oxidative damage, therefore promoting renal health.

The herb astragalus, which has a long history in traditional Chinese medicine, is well known for strengthening the immune system.

By strengthening the immune system, possibly preventing infections, and lowering the risk of problems that could affect renal function, it may improve overall kidney health. Astragalus helps protect the kidneys from any harm by enhancing immunological resilience.

There are other choices to consider among other vital herbs for kidney health. Certain herbs, such as ginger and parsley, are well-known for their diuretic qualities, which encourage the flow of pee and help the body rid itself of waste.

Others, including marshmallow root and juniper berries, have long been used to treat urinary tract problems and promote kidney function.

Kidney health may be preserved by incorporating these vital herbs into a conscious, well-rounded wellness regimen. Before incorporating these herbs into one's regimen, it is imperative to speak with a healthcare provider, especially for people who are taking medication or have pre-existing medical conditions. These herbs can be used in conjunction with a healthy lifestyle that includes eating a balanced meal and staying well hydrated to support and nurture kidney function over the long run.

CHAPTER 5
INCORPORATING HERBS INTO YOUR LIFESTYLE

For generations, herbs have been an integral part of traditional medicine and wellness regimens, providing a natural and comprehensive approach to well-being. Using herbal teas and infusions in your everyday routine is one of the most well-liked ways to include herbs.

These drinks offer several health advantages in addition to a pleasant sensory experience.

Herbal teas, such as those infused with peppermint or chamomile, are well-known for their sedative qualities, which facilitate relaxation and improve digestion. Contrarily, infusions entail steeping herbs in hot water for an extended period to extract more potent chemicals and enhance their therapeutic benefits.

Many people also decide to include herbal supplements in their daily routine in addition to herbal drinks.

These supplements, which are available in a variety of forms such as powders, tinctures, and capsules, provide a practical means of obtaining the concentrated health benefits of particular herbs. Herbal supplements can be customized to address a variety of health needs, such as immune support, stress alleviation, or better sleep.

 But before incorporating herbal supplements into your regimen, it's imperative to speak with a healthcare provider. Individual health concerns and drug interactions need to be taken into account.

Another way to incorporate herbs into your lifestyle is through dietary adjustments, with a particular emphasis on kidney health. Herbs with a reputation for promoting kidney function include dandelion root and parsley. Including these herbs in your diet—either as garnishes or added to salads—can improve your kidneys' general health. In addition, consuming less sodium and drinking plenty of water are complementary dietary approaches that support the best possible kidney function in concert with herbal components.

Experimenting with herbal recipes can be a tasty and inventive method for people who love cooking to improve the nutritional value and flavor of their meals. Herbs like basil, rosemary, and thyme offer a multitude of possible health advantages in addition to enhancing the flavor profile of food. Herbs can improve general wellness and increase the nutritional content of your meals with their anti-inflammatory and antioxidant-rich ingredients.

There are many ways to include herbs into your lifestyle, such as the soothing ritual of making herbal teas, the specific health benefits of supplements, dietary changes for particular health objectives, and the experimentation with herbal recipes in the kitchen. A holistic approach to well-being that acknowledges the connections between mental and physical health as well as the colorful flavors that herbs add to our lives can be fostered by adopting these practices. A lasting and pleasurable integration of herbs into your daily routine is ensured by striking a balance that corresponds with your unique health needs and preferences as you begin this journey.

CHAPTER 6
LIFESTYLE AND DIETARY RECOMMENDATIONS

For kidney health to be at its best, drinking enough of water is essential. For the kidneys to effectively filter waste and poisons out of the bloodstream, an adequate intake of fluids is necessary.

Drinking enough water encourages the dilution of compounds that may otherwise cause kidney stones and urinary tract infections.

This helps avoid these problems from occurring. People should make an effort to drink enough water throughout the day. Although this varies from person to person, it's generally advised to aim for eight 8-ounce glasses of water every day.

A straightforward method of determining one's level of hydration is to look at the color of their urine; a pale-yellow color indicates adequate hydration.

Another essential component of a healthy lifestyle that supports kidney function is regular exercise. Engaging in physical activity lowers the risk of renal disease by promoting cardiovascular health and assisting with blood pressure regulation. Regular exercise also helps with weight control because obesity increases the risk of renal issues. Exercise also enhances general well-being by strengthening the immune system and enhancing mental health, both of which tangentially assist kidney function.

A balanced diet is essential for preventing kidney disease. Essential nutrients can be obtained without taxing the kidneys by eating a diet high in fruits, vegetables, whole grains, and lean meats. Moderate sodium consumption is recommended since high salt intake can lead to fluid retention and hypertension, both of which put stress on the kidneys. It's crucial to keep an eye on your protein intake, particularly if you already have renal disease. Eating too much protein might make your situation worse.

Dietary suggestions can be more specifically tailored to meet the needs and health conditions of each individual by speaking with a trained dietitian or healthcare expert.

One proactive way to maintain kidney health is to stay away from kidney irritants.

Tobacco and excessive alcohol consumption are two substances that can harm the kidneys and accelerate the onset or progression of renal disease. Kidney cancer risk has been associated with smoking in particular. Since nephrotoxic pharmaceuticals, such as nonsteroidal anti-inflammatory drugs (NSAIDs), can damage the kidneys over time, it's also important to limit your intake of these chemicals.

It's critical to understand the possible negative effects of prescription drugs and to seek advice from medical specialists while looking into other possibilities.

To sum up, maintaining kidney health and preventing kidney disease requires a lifestyle that emphasizes being hydrated, getting regular exercise, and eating a balanced diet while avoiding renal stresses. These dietary and lifestyle suggestions operate as preventative steps to protect one of the body's most important organs, guaranteeing lifespan and optimal performance. People are urged to make well-informed decisions, get expert assistance when necessary, and develop lifestyle behaviors that promote general well-being, which includes kidney health.

CHAPTER 7
CASE STUDIES AND SUCCESS STORIES

Real-world experiences with herbal medicines are becoming a fascinating area of study in the field of alternative medicine. One interesting case study addresses the treatment of persistent pain with a traditional herbal medication.

A patient who was unable to find relief from chronic back pain with conventional therapies turned to natural remedies. With the use of a specially prepared concoction of anti-inflammatory herbs, the patient's discomfort was much reduced, and their general health improved. This instance highlights the potential of herbal medicines to offer workable substitutes for people looking for all-encompassing solutions to health issues.

Positive results and testimonials increase the effectiveness of herbal medicines in a variety of health scenarios.

Take the example of a person who struggled with sleeplessness and found relief with herbal drinks and supplements. This firsthand account clarifies the effectiveness of specific herbs in fostering calm and enhancing the caliber of sleep.

These stories not only demonstrate the customized character of herbal therapies but also motivate those who are looking for natural remedies for common health problems.

More broadly, success stories in herbal medicine frequently cover cultural and traditional practices in addition to personal experiences.

Communities with a long history of using herbal treatments have a wealth of testimonies.

For example, a community in a far-off place might demonstrate the long-lasting effectiveness of herbal remedies that have been passed down through the years to heal common illnesses.

These personal accounts offer insightful perspectives on the long-term assimilation of herbal treatments into social and cultural contexts.

In addition, there are success tales involving herbal medicines in the skincare field.

People with chronic skin diseases have frequently seen alleviation from their symptoms by using herbal mixtures. Herbal treatments offer an appealing option for people looking for kinder, natural solutions, whether they are treating eczema, acne, or other skin conditions.

Not only do the testimonials in this area validate the efficiency of the products, but they also provide direction for others as they embark on their skincare journey.

Finally, actual experiences with herbal treatments capture a multitude of positive tales that highlight the adaptability and effectiveness of these natural remedies. The stories surrounding herbal treatments construct a narrative of holistic well-being, ranging from cultural customs to skincare advances, and from controlling chronic pain to encouraging peaceful sleep.

These case studies and testimonies help influence attitudes and cultivate a more thorough comprehension of the possible advantages provided by herbal treatments as people continue to investigate and adopt alternative health techniques.

CHAPTER 8
INTEGRATING WESTERN AND HERBAL APPROACHES
Collaboration with Healthcare Professionals

Promoting cooperation between practitioners in the Western and herbal fields is a crucial part of combining the two approaches to healing.

Gaining a thorough grasp of a patient's health requires acknowledging the advantages and disadvantages of each system. It is imperative that Western medical professionals, including doctors and herbalists, practice open communication and mutual respect. This partnership encourages knowledge sharing and an integrated strategy that maximizes the advantages of both conventional and herbal care. When medical professionals collaborate, they can design individualized treatment programs that cater to each patient's particular requirements and preferences, which will ultimately improve the standard of care provided.

Alternative Medicines

Accepting the idea of complementary therapy is necessary to integrate Western and herbal techniques. Practitioners can see the possible synergies that result from mixing herbal therapies with Western medical techniques, as opposed to seeing these approaches as mutually exclusive.

For example, a patient receiving traditional cancer therapies can also benefit from taking herbal supplements that boost immunity or lessen the negative effects of the medication.

Healthcare professionals can minimize potential side effects and maximize therapeutic outcomes by carefully integrating these alternative therapies. The significance of taking the full person into account and designing treatments to enhance overall well-being is emphasized by this holistic approach.

Handling Drug Interactions

The control of pharmaceutical interactions is an important factor to take into account when integrating Western and herbal therapies.

There is a chance that interactions between the various chemical compositions of herbal medicines and prescription medications could jeopardize patient safety or treatment efficacy. When evaluating and keeping an eye out for possible interactions between prescribed drugs and herbal supplements, healthcare practitioners need to exercise caution.

A full evaluation of the patient's medical history and herbal usage is part of an integrated strategy. In the pursuit of holistic healthcare, practitioners can prioritize patient safety, make well-informed judgments, and make necessary adjustments to treatment plans by remaining knowledgeable about potential interactions.

To sum up, combining Western and herbal medicine requires cooperation between medical experts, awareness of complementary therapies, and careful attention to drug interactions.

By adopting these ideas, healthcare professionals can offer more individualized and thorough treatment that takes into account the advantages of both conventional and herbal therapy.

This integrated strategy could lead to better overall health outcomes for patients and open the door for a more patient-centered and holistic approach to healthcare.

CHAPTER 9
CHALLENGES AND CONTROVERSIES

The absence of solid scientific proof for the effectiveness and security of different herbal treatments is a common grievance voiced by opponents of herbal medicine.

A primary critique centers on the inadequate standardization of herbal products, resulting in discrepancies in terms of composition and efficacy.

Standardized dosages are necessary to generate consistent therapeutic effects; their absence may cause disparities in research outcomes.

Critics contend that the absence of standardization in herbal medicine research presents obstacles to the repeatability of studies, hence impeding the ability to derive dependable findings regarding the efficacy of certain herbal therapies.

The inadequate knowledge of many herbal treatments' mechanisms of action is another point of criticism. While certain herbal components have been the subject of in-depth research, others have not received enough attention, raising concerns about their safety and possible interactions with prescription drugs. Critics frequently stress the need for a thorough investigation to clarify the pharmacological characteristics of herbal remedies, calling for more stringent clinical trials and mechanistic investigations to provide a strong basis for their application.

The debates surrounding the use of herbal medicine are exacerbated by misconceptions and widespread fallacies about it. The idea that because herbal treatments come from natural sources, they are all naturally safe is one common fallacy.

This oversimplification, meanwhile, ignores the reality that nature also contains a variety of dangerous and strong chemicals. Critics contend that people who self-prescribe without thinking about possible side effects or combinations with prescribed medications are encouraged to adopt a slack attitude about the dangers connected with herbal remedies as a result of this misperception.

It is critical to address safety problems in herbal medicine to reduce controversy and promote responsible usage of the product.

One major safety problem is the absence of strict regulatory frameworks and established quality control procedures. The safety of herbal products may be jeopardized by the possibility of contamination, adulteration, or misidentification of herbal substances, according to critics.

To address concerns regarding variable product quality and safety, it is imperative to establish and enforce comprehensive quality control systems that guarantee the authenticity and purity of herbal medicines.

In addition, concerns over the proper education and training of healthcare workers are brought up by the incorporation of herbal medicine into traditional healthcare systems.

Critics contend that a lack of awareness regarding herbal medicines among medical professionals could result in poor patient counseling, possible interactions between herbs and drugs, and delays in necessary medical interventions.

To tackle these issues, it is necessary to provide thorough training programs for medical professionals that will improve their knowledge of herbal remedies and allow them to make well-informed decisions while caring for patients.

There are still issues and debates regarding the use of herbal medicine in healthcare settings because of its negative connotations, false beliefs, and safety concerns. To address these difficulties and promote a more informed and responsible use of herbal treatments, rigorous scientific research, standardization of herbal products, and improved public and healthcare professional education are essential.

CHAPTER 10
FUTURE DIRECTIONS IN HERBAL KIDNEY HEALTH
Research and Findings Continue

Research and discoveries in the field of herbal kidney health are booming and have great potential for the future. Scientists and researchers are exploring the complex mechanisms that underlie how different herbal treatments affect kidney function. Investigating the molecular mechanisms, bioactive ingredients, and combined effects of herbal formulations are all part of this. Extensive clinical trials are being conducted to assess the effectiveness and safety of various herbal remedies for kidney health. As technology develops, scientists are using cutting-edge methods to understand the complex relationships between herbal medicines and renal physiology, including proteomics, metabolomics, and genomes.

The ongoing advancement of research in this area leads to a deeper comprehension of the possible advantages of herbal remedies for renal health maintenance.

Possible Innovations

Potential advances in the field of herbal kidney health require a multidisciplinary approach that incorporates empirical data, traditional knowledge, and state-of-the-art scientific approaches. Finding new bioactive molecules derived from herbs with nephroprotective qualities is one intriguing option.

These substances might exhibit distinct mechanisms of action, focusing on particular cellular pathways related to renal function and minimizing harm. Furthermore, developments in herbal formulations and delivery systems are being investigated to improve therapeutic results and bioavailability. To fully realize the promise of herbal treatments, modern researchers and practitioners of traditional medicine must work together.

The idea of incorporating evidence-based herbal therapies into conventional healthcare procedures is becoming more likely as advancements are made, providing fresh approaches to managing kidney health.

The Changing Face of Complementary Medicine

Herbal medicine is seeing a dynamic transformation as healthcare shifts toward individualized and integrative approaches are taking place. This evolution can be seen in the context of kidney health in the investigation of customized herbal therapies that take into account individual differences in genetics, lifestyle, and environmental factors. An increasing number of people are seeing the benefits of integrative approaches—which blend traditional medical care with herbal remedies—as supplemental methods of maximizing renal health.

Furthermore, to guarantee repeatability and safety, standardization and quality control of herbal products are becoming crucial. Attitudes toward holistic approaches to kidney health are changing as a result of the public's and healthcare professionals' rising acceptance of herbal therapy. Herbal medicine will become a valuable and evidence-based part of renal health management only if rigorous scientific study, interdisciplinary collaboration, and education continue as the area develops.

In conclusion, continuing research projects, the hunt for possible discoveries, and the changing field of herbal medicine describe the future paths in herbal kidney health. The possibility of implementing evidence-based herbal therapies into conventional healthcare practices is becoming more and more real as our comprehension of the intricate relationships between herbs and renal physiology expands.

 The key to realizing the complete benefits of herbal treatments for kidney health lies in their synergy with contemporary scientific methodology. This opens up new avenues in the search for holistic and individualized approaches to renal well-being.

CONCLUSION

It is necessary to summarize the main ideas covered in this discussion. The voyage undertaken has covered a wide range of ideas, exploring the nuances of topics from science and technology to philosophy and human behavior.

A thorough comprehension of the complex nature of our universe is revealed by this investigation. The interdependence of these various domains highlights the complexity inherent in the modern environment.

The quick speed of invention and discovery has been a major theme in the fields of science and technology.

These disciplines are always changing, which forces us to adjust and welcome change and creates an atmosphere where possibilities are never-ending. Critical analysis of the effects of technology development on ethics, the environment, and society has prompted us to consider the responsible use and advancement of these potent instruments.

Contemplation of the nature of reality and existence itself has been prompted by the study of philosophical notions. From conversations about awareness to moral conundrums, the philosophical trip has stimulated reflection and discussion, pushing readers to challenge presumptions and have thoughtful conversations. A comprehensive understanding of the human condition has been made possible by the nexus of philosophy and science, where existential reflection and logical investigation collide.

Examining the subtleties of psychology and human behavior has helped to clarify the nuances and reasons that shape our interactions.

A complex understanding of human nature has been revealed via research on cognitive processes and the effects of social systems. We are reminded of the humanistic elements that cut over disciplinary lines as we acknowledge the importance of empathy and compassion in navigating the complex web of connections.

Encouragement for more research and intellectual curiosity is crucial as readers make their way through the provided ideas.

 The ideas discussed here provide a springboard for further investigation in the never-ending pursuit of knowledge. An open mind and a desire to learn are priceless in the ever-evolving world of ideas and information. We want all readers to follow their intellectual interests, participate in meaningful discussions, and add to the body of information that helps to shape our perception of the world.

The convergence of these disparate ideas essentially highlights the depth of intellectual inquiry.

As we consider the main ideas raised, let's not see them separately but rather as interwoven threads that make up a larger picture of comprehension. Readers are encouraged to actively participate in the continuing conversation that advances humanity, rather than just absorbing knowledge. By doing this, we all add to the body of knowledge that humans possess and keep deciphering the mysteries that surround our existence.